Mindful Scrolling Mastery

A Guide to Breaking Doomscrolling Habits

TABLE OF CONTENT

Introduction

Are you prone to doomscrolling? Do you frequently check your social media accounts to see what negative or gloomy news has been posted recently? A somewhat recent word, "doomscrolling," refers to a bad behavior that has become more prevalent since the advent of smartphones and social media.

People read a great deal about various topics every day, such as the most recent COVID-19 outbreak, the status of their nation's economy, natural disasters, global warming, the possibility of war, murders and other crimes, and more.

These days, there are a plethora of things that could give you a bad experience. The most recent school shootings in the US and the seemingly unchecked proliferation of

COVID-19 and its derivatives are topics covered in the press every day. There is a plethora of information available to you if you wish to instill negativity in yourself.

Breaking terrible news is not a standard practice. There was negative news reported in newspapers and on television before the Internet and social media (this is still going on now). It is detrimental to your mental health to read and listen to these negative news items regularly. However, it's a habit that can be broken.

We'll go in-depth on doomscrolling, also known as "doomsurfing," in this special report and see how it can be detrimental to your mental health. Next, we'll share how you can break free from this bad behavior and adopt positive, empowered ones in its place.

These powerful routines will improve your quality of life. Okay, how about we move forward with this? We will explain what doomscrolling is in the next section.

Chapter 1:
What Doomscrolling Really Is

Our favorite way to describe doomscrolling is as "obsessively looking for and absorbing bad news." Doomscrolling is a habit that a person will stick with even after realizing it makes them anxious.

You have most likely been developing the habit of doomscrolling for years. Even though you know it hurts, you can't seem to stop doing it. You constantly have to have your fill of terrible news, and you'll do whatever it takes to obtain it.

It's thought that Twitter is where the word "doomscrolling" first appeared. Because of the wiring in our brains, everyone is prone to this harmful behavior. Psychologists are aware that when we consider a situation to be threatening, our brains will automatically focus on it. We have a survival instinct that includes this.

We are Programmed for Survival

Your brain is constantly examining your surroundings to identify any possible threats, even though you are usually unaware of this. Threats to your survival rank highest on the priority list, and your brain prioritizes these over other issues.

We all want to survive, therefore this is a good thing. The issue lies in the fact that, even in situations where we are not in danger, our brains tend to choose negative narratives over-optimistic ones.

When it comes to our protection and safety, we're never done searching for more information. We have to discover better answers if we are unable to find the information we need or if there is contradicting data, so we keep searching for bad news.

Soon enough, you'll be searching through your social media accounts for any negative updates. Your happiness is being negatively impacted by the negativity cycle you have entered. Do you know any persons that seem to be negative all the time? They are everywhere, and doomscrolling may or may not be partial to fault.

Our prehistoric forebears were alert for negative news at all times. To protect themselves, they needed to know if any predators were in the area. For them, this information was more valuable than freshwater or food sources.

Don't Feel Bad About Being a Doomscroller

We don't want you to feel horrible if you often engage in doomscrolling. These days, most people do it. Every human has a natural curiosity for new things. If this information can increase our chances of survival and keep us safe, then it is vital to us.

However, you should be aware that compulsive doom-scrolling can not only make you feel bad about yourself, but it can also cost you valuable time. Are you having trouble finishing anything because you can't stop looking for the worst news? Isn't it preferable to utilize the time you would normally spend doomscrolling for something constructive?

It's not easy to Break the Doomscrolling Habit but it is Possible

Although you won't be able to kick the habit of doomscrolling easily, it is doable. Since almost everyone owns a smartphone these days, it is all too simple to rapidly check social media and absorb all the negative news you could ever desire from various websites and news applications.

However, don't let this convince you that you can't overcome your tendency to doomscrolling. This unique study will show you that there are more constructive things you can do to break the habit of doomscrolling. Your life will be significantly improved by these new experiences, and you will have a far more optimistic view of it.

You need to understand the potential harm that doomscrolling might cause to you daily before we discuss how to break the practice. Most likely, you are unaware that these things are occurring to you.

We'll talk about the potential effects of doomscrolling on your life in the following section.

Chapter 2:
The Possible Impact of Doomscrolling on your Life

Now, let's get a little technical and explain how your brain functions. When you expose your "lizard brain" to unfavorable information, it becomes active. Your brain contains a structure called the "amygdala," a group of cells located close to the base of the brain.

This area of your brain is crucial because it sets off your body's defense mechanisms if something in your surroundings poses a threat. This will make you actively search your surroundings for danger when it activates.

Fight or Flight Mode

We should all be thankful that your brain is constantly trying to warn you to stay vigilant if it feels like your life is in danger. Additionally, it keeps us from making foolish decisions like running into oncoming traffic or leaping from towering buildings.

Your limbic system kicks your body into fight-or-flight mode when it detects danger. This implies that you will either flee the scene as quickly as possible or protect yourself by standing your ground and engaging in combat.

You have the fastest reaction times while you're in fight or flight mode. This will assist you in escaping a potentially fatal situation. Your pulse rate quickens dramatically, and you may become so terrified that you freeze.

While your body is in fight-or-flight mode, you have little chance of resting.

Doomscrolling is hard-wired in your Brain

Humans will always be able to respond to threats in an adaptive fashion. We have evolved as a species to do whatever it takes to live long and prosper. It is perfectly normal for us to be constantly on the lookout for danger.

The media and social media corporations are fully aware of this innate tendency. As they say, "bad news sells newspapers," and this is true. It was inevitable that doomscrolling would catch on with so many people since there was always negative stuff available and it was made available to everyone on social media.

Social media firms want you to share all the horrible things you come across with your pals and to never stop reading through your newsfeed. They want you to spend as much time as possible staring at your screen. On social media, there are a lot of opportunities for you to find terrible news, and once you do, it can be hard to quit since there is so much of it to take in.

The coronavirus outbreak made people more inclined to doomsday. For all of us, it has been a trying moment, and many individuals were forced to absorb all of the negative news. People would inevitably be browsing for the newest dark news regarding COVID-19 because it poses a threat to our survival.

We don't need Bad News to Survive

In modern life, terrible news is not as necessary as it was for our ancient predecessors to survive. If you search for it, you can now get negative news from all around the world. In actuality, this news has relatively little impact on our lives.

We do not need to keep scrolling down to get more awful news. It is something that individuals in today's world choose to do, not something that threatens our survival. Even though we don't have to hear this awful news, doing so can still be detrimental to our physical and mental well-being.

Since COVID-19 poses a serious risk, it is bound to activate our amygdala. However, many became extremely compulsive because of the negative news surrounding it. Your perspectives will be negatively altered if you just hear terrible news all the time.

Doomscrolling can Intensify Irrational Fear

You may come to feel that the world is much more hazardous than it truly is if you are always doomscrolling. Your level of anxiety and concern increases as you continue to doomscroll. It may be necessary for you to actively search for bad things, which will only make matters worse.

Doomscrolling too much can make you feel hopeless and like you're headed for disaster, which is why it's unhealthy. It's possible for your unreasonable concerns to get stronger and for new ones to emerge. It can amplify your brain's pessimistic bias, making you continuously on the lookout for new evidence that the world is a terrible place.

Doomscrolling is a Time Stealer

Nothing is more valuable than time. No matter how wealthy you are, you cannot purchase more of it. Doomscrolling also has the significant drawback of taking up a lot of your time. According to a New York Times report, Americans have been staring at their computer or smartphone screens for half as long as before the outbreak.

Consider all the beneficial things you could accomplish with the time you squandered.

You may spend more time with your loved ones and friends and complete a lot more work. In life, these things are significantly more significant than social media.

Doomscrolling can Negatively Impact your Mental and Physical Health

The detrimental effects that doomscrolling can have on your physical and mental well-being are far worse than just being a time waster. Anxiety, tension, and despair can all rise with excessive doomscrolling. You should stay away from these items at all costs as they have the potential to damage your life.

Furthermore, doomscrolling can lead to a variety of physical health issues. An increasing number of people these days are experiencing headaches, insomnia, tummy problems, increased muscle tension, and more.

Receiving bad news all the time can lead to serious anxiety disorders as well as several physical health problems. All of this can result in depression because of the illogical worry that you are always in danger when you are not. Those who are constantly on the lookout for bad news may even exhibit hostile and aggressive conduct because they think there is always a risk.

Many people enjoy doing their doomscrolling during the late hours of the night, which interferes with their sleep. When they do want to sleep at last, the doomscrolling can make it difficult for them to do so. They have a sense of unease about their surroundings, which can lead to elevated tension and anxiety. This makes finding more bad news more necessary.

It can become a Vicious Cycle

If your level of doomscrolling has left you in a poor mood, you'll probably be extremely sensitive to further emotionally upsetting terrible news. It may amplify your illogical anxieties and heighten your anxiety. You thus have a greater need for more unfavorable information.

These days, there is so much terrible news that it can make you feel more anxious. Although you are eager to stay current on everything, you are unable to accomplish so.

Individuals simply can't get enough of this bad knowledge because they genuinely think it is essential to their survival.

They are forced to never stop looking for solutions, which sends them into a vicious cycle that is very hard to escape. Depression and anxiety may shortly follow. If you start to feel nervous, you think that learning more would give you back control. The only way to break the vicious cycle is to overcome your ingrained tendencies.

Breaking the Habit of Doomscrolling Will Be Difficult

In this report, we want to be as realistic as we can. You should be aware that breaking your habit of doomscrolling will need a great deal of self-control. You can overcome doomscrolling, even though there are no quick fixes.

To combat your want to keep doomscrolling, you'll need to be determined to quit, as well as have strong attention and energy. This implies that to avoid doomscrolling without thinking, you must become more self-aware. Replacing the doomscrolling behavior with an empowering one is the most effective method to overcome it.

To improve your life, you must establish a more optimistic daily routine. The coronavirus pandemic has caused many people to lose faith in humanity. They believe they no longer have control over their lives as a result of the pandemic. This is something none of us have ever encountered before. For some, it has caused extreme anxiety.

Research Studies Prove the Negative Impact of Bad News

Numerous studies have established a connection between poor mental health and frequent exposure to negative news. These days, you can always find negative news online. Before social media and the Internet, you had to watch the news on TV to get your daily fix of negativity.

These days, it is quite simple to take in a lot of terrible news. People are becoming more stressed as a result, which raises the prevalence of anxiety and depression. You most likely didn't set out to be a doomscroller; instead, the abundance of unfavorable information made you one.

Psychologists refer to compulsive doomsayers as having an "intolerance of uncertainty." This is the reason why doom-scrolling is such a hard habit to stop. Even when they hear bad news, some people can't stop wanting to know what's going on in the world.

A study was done to find out how participants responded to both good and negative headlines. What impact may a favorable or negative headline have on the participants' attitudes in the study? Thirty volunteers in total were split up into three groups for the study.

The first group received mostly good news, the second received a mix of both good and terrible news, and the final group received mostly poor news. They assessed each participant's mood both before and after the trial started. The study's conclusion did not come as a shock to anyone.

Compared to the participants in the other two groups, everyone in the third group— which had been receiving terrible news constantly—was in a more heightened state of fear and anxiety. It was discovered that those in the group who received negative news tended to worry far more about their concerns.

This implies that you are more likely to have anxiety about things other than what you are reading if you are continuously reading doomsday articles and terrible news. Most likely, you'll begin to concentrate on the aspects of your life that you find stressful and that you believe are out of your control.

Technology Compounds the Problem

Though it's a great thing, doomscrolling is made worse by modern technology. These days, anyone can use social media to look up information on any topic and read all the negative news they want. People always have access to terrible news because they always carry their smartphones with them.

Search engines and social media platforms have sophisticated algorithms that learn about your interests and present you with more of the same, which exacerbates the issue even further. They continuously give you the material you desire because they want you to be as involved on their platforms as possible.

As a result, even if it wasn't your intention, you will continuously be presented with unfavorable stuff. Because you are exposed to this stuff daily, it becomes increasingly difficult to avoid it.

To kick the habit of doomscrolling, you will have to fight off search engines and your social network accounts. Regaining control over the information you consume online will require effort on your part. It will be quite beneficial to alter the content that you read and seek on social media.

You should be aware that the preferences that search engines and social media algorithms use to determine your preferences may take some time to change.

Even if you decide to stop doomscrolling, you will continue to see unfavorable stuff on these platforms for a long.

However, the willpower and perseverance needed to quit doomscrolling will undoubtedly be worthwhile. Your anxiety and stress levels will eventually decrease, and you'll feel a lot better about your life overall. Choosing to stop doomscrolling is the best one you can make.

We'll talk about how to stop doomscrolling in the future part.

How to Break Free from Doomscrolling

You're going to need to create a new daily routine if you want to stop doomscrolling.

You must make a shift in your life's course to absorb less negative news stories. You will need to do this by applying constant effort to take back control of your life and by staying focused on your goals.

There are many advantages to quitting your practice of doomscrolling. You'll feel so much better about your life once you start implementing new, empowered rituals to replace your constant search for bad news. Additionally, you'll feel less anxious and stressed and regain control of your life.

Minimize your Sources of Bad News

There are a lot of locations to find terrible news, and if you are a frequent user of many sources, you can minimize the number of websites you visit to get a head start on quitting doomscrolling. As a result, you will be exposed to less negative news every day.

Assume in the meantime that you are doomscrolling and visiting eight different websites. You'll probably keep receiving the same terrible news, which will just encourage your habit. You can progressively lessen the anxiety triggers that come from repeatedly seeing the same news by cutting down on the number of websites you frequent.

You should also keep a careful eye on the emotional toll that receiving negative news takes on you. You should stop receiving unfavorable news from that source as soon as possible if it is making you anxious and giving you ongoing trouble. Locating positive news websites to take the place of negative ones is a smart move.

Take a Vacation from Electronics

Decide to put your smartphone and computer away for a while. If you find another way to replace the hole in your life, doing this is rather simple. Inform followers on your social media pages that you will no longer be answering every message right away.

It's simple to switch off your computer or store your smartphone in a hard-to-reach location. Get an inexpensive phone that can't be used to browse the internet or install apps if you're worried about missing calls and texts. Any unreasonable anxieties will subside if you take brief vacations from your electronics.

Take little pauses at first, and then progressively increase this. Life is more than just the Internet and social media. You will be able to collect your thoughts and consider what you are doing when you take your pauses.

Ask yourself Questions about your Doomscrolling Habit

You can make progress in kicking your doomscrolling habit by asking yourself the correct questions. The following inquiries will prompt you to consider your actions more carefully:

Is the stuff I'm reading helping me or is it simply making me feel pessimistic?

When I receive the awful news, how do I feel?

Do I have to stop doing other pleasant activities because I'm doomscrolling?

Does doing my doomscrolling make me more hostile and irrational?

Am I making sure the unpleasant news I'm reading is accurate before allowing it to impact me?

Am I spreading unfavorable rumors to others without confirming them?

You must provide truthful answers to each of these inquiries. If you tell yourself lies, you will not get very far in breaking your doomscrolling habit.

We want to be clear that breaking up with your doomscrolling habit does not entail that you should never stay up to date with significant events taking place around the globe. We advise you to verify that the information is accurate and pertinent to you by challenging it.

You can steer clear of a lot of the bad feelings that will impede your progress in life by challenging the food you are consuming in this manner. You will find it difficult to comprehend both your surroundings and the people in them, for instance, if your doomscrolling causes you to feel frightened and enraged.

Increasing your Awareness is a Critical

We explained before that our innate desire to doomsday is a result of the way our brains are hardwired. You will never be able to break the habit if you punish yourself for this. Commit to becoming more conscious of the information you are consuming in its place.

Remember that the globe has come a long way since our ancient ancestors lived here. In modern life, bad news is not necessary for them to survive the way it did for them. The likelihood of a troop of lions attempting to attack you in your neighborhood is very low.

Gaining more self-awareness will assist you in putting this all into context. Most of the bad stuff you read when doomscrolling is irrelevant to you and of little use to you. You were just naturally drawn to search for it, and you may overcome this inclination by practicing self-awareness.

Preserving your time and mental space is a wise move. To do this, recognize how much information you take in each day and categorize everything. Thus, you may group the data you take into the following categories:

I must be aware of this.

I'm curious about this.

You don't have to tell me this.

You'll be able to tell how much information you take in is a sign of your doomscrolling habit after a short while of doing this. After that, you can take steps to get rid of the material that doesn't apply to your life.

Evaluating your emotions while you are taking in information is another technique to become more self-aware. Stop absorbing such material if it is causing you any tension or anxiety.

You won't always find accuracy in what you read online, especially on social networking platforms. Sometimes, even well-known news websites make mistakes. Making every effort to ensure that the information you are consuming is accurate can undoubtedly help you.

You should only take in information that is supported by facts, not just opinions. Opinions are not reliable and are frequently incorrect. After making every effort to confirm the truth of the information you are consuming, do not react to it.

Conclusion

You now understand the reasons for doomscrolling and the detrimental effects it can have on your life. Now is the moment to stop your doomscrolling habit and take action. There is no miracle remedy for doomscrolling in this report—it does not exist.

The good news is that you can overcome doomscrolling, but it will require determination and constant effort. Recall that not doomscrolling is also a habit and that doomscrolling is merely a habit. Replacing your doomscrolling habit will require patience and perseverance, but you can succeed.

Being self-aware is essential to escaping the doomscrolling cycle. To be fully aware of the stuff you are consuming daily, you need to work on developing your self-awareness. Take responsibility for your actions and start watching what you eat.

It will require self-control to do this because it is quite simple to browse through websites and consume damaging, negative stuff. Here, remember the wider picture. Remind yourself that consuming negative stuff will make you feel more stressed and nervous when you are tempted to start doomscrolling again—which is quite likely to happen at first.

Additionally, remind yourself that doomscrolling degrades your life's quality. Instead of doomscrolling, you could be spending time with your loved ones and friends, among other beneficial activities.

You can choose not to get news alerts if you have already opted in. Make a deliberate decision about the stuff you will absorb. With intention, you'll be forced to employ parts of your brain that aren't utilized for mindless scrolling.

We wish you every success breaking free from doomscrolling.

Essential Resources
What is doomscrolling and how to stop it

https://www.health.com/mind-body/what-is-doomscrolling

Why doomscrolling is bad for your mental health

https://www.psychologytoday.com/us/blog/i-hear-you/202011/here-s-why-doomscrolling-is-so-bad-your-mental-health

3 apps to help you stop doomscrolling

https://techunwrapped.com/3-apps-to-stop-doomscrolling-2021/

6 tips to stop doomscrolling

https://happiful.com/tips-to-stop-doomscrolling/